# Emergency Airway Management Logbook

Name:

Start Date:

Book No.:

▮ Please complete for all bag-mask ventilation (BMV) with bag-valve-mask (BVM)

▮ Please complete for all use of essential adjuncts

▮ Please complete for all use of extra-glottic devices

▮ Please complete for all ET intubation attempts

▮ Please complete for all use of needle/surgical airway

▮ Please complete for all use of other clinical skills

Text © Jamie Todd 2019

All rights reserved. Without limiting the rights under copyright reserved above, no part of this publication may be reproduced, stored in or introduced into a retrieval system, or transmitted, in any form or by any means (electronic, mechanical, photocopying, recording or otherwise) without the prior written permission of the publisher of this book.

The information presented in this book is accurate and current to the best of the authors' knowledge.

The authors and publisher, however, make no guarantee as to, and assume no responsibility for, the correctness, sufficiency or completeness of such information or recommendation.

Printing history
This edition first published 2019 (reprinted 2019, 2022 and 2024)

The authors and publisher welcome feedback from the users of this book. Please contact the publisher:

Class Professional Publishing,
The Exchange, Express Park, Bristol Road, Bridgwater TA6 4RR
Telephone: 01278 427 826
Email: info@class.co.uk
www.classprofessional.co.uk

Class Professional Publishing is an imprint of Class Publishing Ltd
A CIP catalogue record for this book is available from the British Library

Cover design by Hybert Design Limited
Cover image from Pre-Hospital Care Consultancy
Designed and typeset by Class Professional Publishing
Printed in the UK by Hobbs the Printers Ltd, Totton, Hampshire

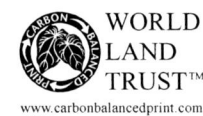

www.carbonbalancedprint.com
CBP2250

# Introduction

This logbook is designed to allow Pre-Hospital and Emergency Care clinicians of all grades to quickly and easily maintain a record of airway skills performed in order to assist in proving competence where required. It allows for rapid after action logging of pertinent details for a number of skills performed in limited numbers. Please use the codes below to aid in filling in your logbook:

- AA – Airway reassessed and open
- AB – Adult BVM
- AV – Assisted ventilation
- BC – Bilateral chest rise
- BS – Breath sounds
- CE – Capnometric $EtCO_2$
- CI – Can't intubate, can't oxygenate
- CL1 – Cormack-Lehane grade 1 view
- CL2 – Cormack-Lehane grade 2 view
- CL3 – Cormack-Lehane grade 3 view
- CL4 – Cormack-Lehane grade 4 view
- CO – Colorimetric $EtCO_2$
- CP – Expected clinical pathway
- DM – DL with mac size?
- DS – DL with straight blade size?
- IG – iGel
- IT – Intubating LMA
- LL – LMA type 2nd gen
- LM – LMA classic
- LT – Laryngeal tube
- MA – To maintain airway
- MV – Manual ventilation
- NB – Neonatal BVM
- NC – Needle cricothyrotomy
- NW – Not worked
- OA – Occluded airway
- OC – One person CE grip
- OL – Optical laryngoscope blade size?
- PB – Paediatric BVM
- PO – Pre-oxygenation
- RS – RSI
- SC – Surgical cricothyrotomy
- TA – To open airway
- TC – Two person CE grip
- TE – Two person TE grip
- VL – Video laryngoscope blade size?
- WE – Waveform $EtCO_2$
- WO – Worked
- VV – Ventilator ventilation

# How To Use This Book

Please refer to the below examples for ways in which you may wish to use this logbook:

BMV with BVM:

| Date | Persons* | Case | Age | Indication* | Bag size* | Tidal vol | Confirm* |
|------|----------|------|-----|-------------|-----------|-----------|----------|
| 1/7/18 | OC/TE | 123 | 18 | AV/MV | AB/PB | 400 | BC |

Essential adjuncts:

| Date | OP/NP | Case | Age | Indication* | Size | NP side? | Confirm* |
|------|-------|------|-----|-------------|------|----------|----------|
| 1/7/18 | OP/NP | 123 | 18 | MA | 7x2 | BOTH | BC |

Extra-glottic device:

| Date | EGD type* | Case | Age | Indication* | Size | Attempts | Confirm* |
|------|-----------|------|-----|-------------|------|----------|----------|
| 1/7/18 | IG/LL | 123 | 18 | MA | 4 | 1 | WE |

Endotracheal (ET) intubation:

| Date | INT/ASS | Case | Indication* | DL/VL* | View* | Bougie | Attempts | Confirm* |
|------|---------|------|-------------|--------|-------|--------|----------|----------|
| 1/7/18 | INT/ASS | 123 | MA | DL/VL | 2 | Y | 2 | WE |

Needle / surgical:

| Date | Procedure* | Case | Age | Indication* | Kit used | Outcome* | Confirm* |
|------|------------|------|-----|-------------|----------|----------|----------|
| 9/7/18 | SC | 777 | 35 | OA | Scalpel bougie | WO | WE |

Other clinical skills:

| Date | Skill | Case | Age | Indication* | Site | Kit used | Confirm* |
|------|-------|------|-----|-------------|------|----------|----------|
| 10/7/18 | Chest decomp | 778 | 31 | Pneumothorax | L 2nd IC MCL | ThoraQuik | BS |

## Please complete for all BMV with BVM
(Use codes in index where indicated*)

| Date | Persons* | Case | Age | Indication* | Bag size* | Tidal vol | Confirm* |
|------|----------|------|-----|-------------|-----------|-----------|----------|
|      |          |      |     |             |           |           |          |
|      |          |      |     |             |           |           |          |
|      |          |      |     |             |           |           |          |
|      |          |      |     |             |           |           |          |
|      |          |      |     |             |           |           |          |
|      |          |      |     |             |           |           |          |
|      |          |      |     |             |           |           |          |
|      |          |      |     |             |           |           |          |
|      |          |      |     |             |           |           |          |
|      |          |      |     |             |           |           |          |
|      |          |      |     |             |           |           |          |
|      |          |      |     |             |           |           |          |
|      |          |      |     |             |           |           |          |

## Please complete for all BMV with BVM
(Use codes in index where indicated*)

| Date | Persons* | Case | Age | Indication* | Bag size* | Tidal vol | Confirm* |
|------|----------|------|-----|-------------|-----------|-----------|----------|
|      |          |      |     |             |           |           |          |
|      |          |      |     |             |           |           |          |
|      |          |      |     |             |           |           |          |
|      |          |      |     |             |           |           |          |
|      |          |      |     |             |           |           |          |
|      |          |      |     |             |           |           |          |
|      |          |      |     |             |           |           |          |
|      |          |      |     |             |           |           |          |
|      |          |      |     |             |           |           |          |
|      |          |      |     |             |           |           |          |
|      |          |      |     |             |           |           |          |
|      |          |      |     |             |           |           |          |
|      |          |      |     |             |           |           |          |

## Please complete for all BMV with BVM
(Use codes in index where indicated*)

| Date | Persons* | Case | Age | Indication* | Bag size* | Tidal vol | Confirm* |
|------|----------|------|-----|-------------|-----------|-----------|----------|
|      |          |      |     |             |           |           |          |
|      |          |      |     |             |           |           |          |
|      |          |      |     |             |           |           |          |
|      |          |      |     |             |           |           |          |
|      |          |      |     |             |           |           |          |
|      |          |      |     |             |           |           |          |
|      |          |      |     |             |           |           |          |
|      |          |      |     |             |           |           |          |
|      |          |      |     |             |           |           |          |
|      |          |      |     |             |           |           |          |
|      |          |      |     |             |           |           |          |
|      |          |      |     |             |           |           |          |
|      |          |      |     |             |           |           |          |
|      |          |      |     |             |           |           |          |

## Please complete for all BMV with BVM
(Use codes in index where indicated*)

| Date | Persons* | Case | Age | Indication* | Bag size* | Tidal vol | Confirm* |
|------|----------|------|-----|-------------|-----------|-----------|----------|
|      |          |      |     |             |           |           |          |
|      |          |      |     |             |           |           |          |
|      |          |      |     |             |           |           |          |
|      |          |      |     |             |           |           |          |
|      |          |      |     |             |           |           |          |
|      |          |      |     |             |           |           |          |
|      |          |      |     |             |           |           |          |
|      |          |      |     |             |           |           |          |
|      |          |      |     |             |           |           |          |
|      |          |      |     |             |           |           |          |
|      |          |      |     |             |           |           |          |
|      |          |      |     |             |           |           |          |
|      |          |      |     |             |           |           |          |

## Please complete for all BMV with BVM
(Use codes in index where indicated*)

| Date | Persons* | Case | Age | Indication* | Bag size* | Tidal vol | Confirm* |
|------|----------|------|-----|-------------|-----------|-----------|----------|
|      |          |      |     |             |           |           |          |
|      |          |      |     |             |           |           |          |
|      |          |      |     |             |           |           |          |
|      |          |      |     |             |           |           |          |
|      |          |      |     |             |           |           |          |
|      |          |      |     |             |           |           |          |
|      |          |      |     |             |           |           |          |
|      |          |      |     |             |           |           |          |
|      |          |      |     |             |           |           |          |
|      |          |      |     |             |           |           |          |
|      |          |      |     |             |           |           |          |
|      |          |      |     |             |           |           |          |
|      |          |      |     |             |           |           |          |

## Please complete for all BMV with BVM
(Use codes in index where indicated*)

| Date | Persons* | Case | Age | Indication* | Bag size* | Tidal vol | Confirm* |
|------|----------|------|-----|-------------|-----------|-----------|----------|
|      |          |      |     |             |           |           |          |
|      |          |      |     |             |           |           |          |
|      |          |      |     |             |           |           |          |
|      |          |      |     |             |           |           |          |
|      |          |      |     |             |           |           |          |
|      |          |      |     |             |           |           |          |
|      |          |      |     |             |           |           |          |
|      |          |      |     |             |           |           |          |
|      |          |      |     |             |           |           |          |
|      |          |      |     |             |           |           |          |
|      |          |      |     |             |           |           |          |
|      |          |      |     |             |           |           |          |
|      |          |      |     |             |           |           |          |
|      |          |      |     |             |           |           |          |

## Please complete for all use of essential adjuncts
(Use codes in index where indicated*)

| Date | OP/NP | Case | Age | Indication* | Size | NP side? | Confirm* |
|------|-------|------|-----|-------------|------|----------|----------|
|      |       |      |     |             |      |          |          |
|      |       |      |     |             |      |          |          |
|      |       |      |     |             |      |          |          |
|      |       |      |     |             |      |          |          |
|      |       |      |     |             |      |          |          |
|      |       |      |     |             |      |          |          |
|      |       |      |     |             |      |          |          |
|      |       |      |     |             |      |          |          |
|      |       |      |     |             |      |          |          |
|      |       |      |     |             |      |          |          |
|      |       |      |     |             |      |          |          |
|      |       |      |     |             |      |          |          |
|      |       |      |     |             |      |          |          |

## Please complete for all use of essential adjuncts
(Use codes in index where indicated*)

| Date | OP/NP | Case | Age | Indication* | Size | NP side? | Confirm* |
|------|-------|------|-----|-------------|------|----------|----------|
|      |       |      |     |             |      |          |          |
|      |       |      |     |             |      |          |          |
|      |       |      |     |             |      |          |          |
|      |       |      |     |             |      |          |          |
|      |       |      |     |             |      |          |          |
|      |       |      |     |             |      |          |          |
|      |       |      |     |             |      |          |          |
|      |       |      |     |             |      |          |          |
|      |       |      |     |             |      |          |          |
|      |       |      |     |             |      |          |          |
|      |       |      |     |             |      |          |          |
|      |       |      |     |             |      |          |          |
|      |       |      |     |             |      |          |          |
|      |       |      |     |             |      |          |          |

## Please complete for all use of essential adjuncts
(Use codes in index where indicated*)

| Date | OP/NP | Case | Age | Indication* | Size | NP side? | Confirm* |
|------|-------|------|-----|-------------|------|----------|----------|
|      |       |      |     |             |      |          |          |
|      |       |      |     |             |      |          |          |
|      |       |      |     |             |      |          |          |
|      |       |      |     |             |      |          |          |
|      |       |      |     |             |      |          |          |
|      |       |      |     |             |      |          |          |
|      |       |      |     |             |      |          |          |
|      |       |      |     |             |      |          |          |
|      |       |      |     |             |      |          |          |
|      |       |      |     |             |      |          |          |
|      |       |      |     |             |      |          |          |
|      |       |      |     |             |      |          |          |
|      |       |      |     |             |      |          |          |

## Please complete for all use of essential adjuncts
(Use codes in index where indicated*)

| Date | OP/NP | Case | Age | Indication* | Size | NP side? | Confirm* |
|------|-------|------|-----|-------------|------|----------|----------|
|      |       |      |     |             |      |          |          |
|      |       |      |     |             |      |          |          |
|      |       |      |     |             |      |          |          |
|      |       |      |     |             |      |          |          |
|      |       |      |     |             |      |          |          |
|      |       |      |     |             |      |          |          |
|      |       |      |     |             |      |          |          |
|      |       |      |     |             |      |          |          |
|      |       |      |     |             |      |          |          |
|      |       |      |     |             |      |          |          |
|      |       |      |     |             |      |          |          |
|      |       |      |     |             |      |          |          |
|      |       |      |     |             |      |          |          |

## Please complete for all use of essential adjuncts
(Use codes in index where indicated*)

| Date | OP/NP | Case | Age | Indication* | Size | NP side? | Confirm* |
|------|-------|------|-----|-------------|------|----------|----------|
|      |       |      |     |             |      |          |          |
|      |       |      |     |             |      |          |          |
|      |       |      |     |             |      |          |          |
|      |       |      |     |             |      |          |          |
|      |       |      |     |             |      |          |          |
|      |       |      |     |             |      |          |          |
|      |       |      |     |             |      |          |          |
|      |       |      |     |             |      |          |          |
|      |       |      |     |             |      |          |          |
|      |       |      |     |             |      |          |          |
|      |       |      |     |             |      |          |          |
|      |       |      |     |             |      |          |          |
|      |       |      |     |             |      |          |          |
|      |       |      |     |             |      |          |          |

## Please complete for all use of essential adjuncts
(Use codes in index where indicated*)

| Date | OP/NP | Case | Age | Indication* | Size | NP side? | Confirm* |
|------|-------|------|-----|-------------|------|----------|----------|
|      |       |      |     |             |      |          |          |
|      |       |      |     |             |      |          |          |
|      |       |      |     |             |      |          |          |
|      |       |      |     |             |      |          |          |
|      |       |      |     |             |      |          |          |
|      |       |      |     |             |      |          |          |
|      |       |      |     |             |      |          |          |
|      |       |      |     |             |      |          |          |
|      |       |      |     |             |      |          |          |
|      |       |      |     |             |      |          |          |
|      |       |      |     |             |      |          |          |
|      |       |      |     |             |      |          |          |
|      |       |      |     |             |      |          |          |

# Please complete for all use of extra-glottic devices
(Use codes in index where indicated*)

| Date | EGD type* | Case | Age | Indication* | Size | Attempts | Confirm* |
|------|-----------|------|-----|-------------|------|----------|----------|
|      |           |      |     |             |      |          |          |
|      |           |      |     |             |      |          |          |
|      |           |      |     |             |      |          |          |
|      |           |      |     |             |      |          |          |
|      |           |      |     |             |      |          |          |
|      |           |      |     |             |      |          |          |
|      |           |      |     |             |      |          |          |
|      |           |      |     |             |      |          |          |
|      |           |      |     |             |      |          |          |
|      |           |      |     |             |      |          |          |
|      |           |      |     |             |      |          |          |
|      |           |      |     |             |      |          |          |
|      |           |      |     |             |      |          |          |

## Please complete for all use of extra-glottic devices
(Use codes in index where indicated*)

| Date | EGD type* | Case | Age | Indication* | Size | Attempts | Confirm* |
|------|-----------|------|-----|-------------|------|----------|----------|
|      |           |      |     |             |      |          |          |
|      |           |      |     |             |      |          |          |
|      |           |      |     |             |      |          |          |
|      |           |      |     |             |      |          |          |
|      |           |      |     |             |      |          |          |
|      |           |      |     |             |      |          |          |
|      |           |      |     |             |      |          |          |
|      |           |      |     |             |      |          |          |
|      |           |      |     |             |      |          |          |
|      |           |      |     |             |      |          |          |
|      |           |      |     |             |      |          |          |
|      |           |      |     |             |      |          |          |
|      |           |      |     |             |      |          |          |

# Please complete for all use of extra-glottic devices
(Use codes in index where indicated*)

| Date | EGD type* | Case | Age | Indication* | Size | Attempts | Confirm* |
|------|-----------|------|-----|-------------|------|----------|----------|
|      |           |      |     |             |      |          |          |
|      |           |      |     |             |      |          |          |
|      |           |      |     |             |      |          |          |
|      |           |      |     |             |      |          |          |
|      |           |      |     |             |      |          |          |
|      |           |      |     |             |      |          |          |
|      |           |      |     |             |      |          |          |
|      |           |      |     |             |      |          |          |
|      |           |      |     |             |      |          |          |
|      |           |      |     |             |      |          |          |
|      |           |      |     |             |      |          |          |
|      |           |      |     |             |      |          |          |
|      |           |      |     |             |      |          |          |

# Please complete for all use of extra-glottic devices
(Use codes in index where indicated*)

| Date | EGD type* | Case | Age | Indication* | Size | Attempts | Confirm* |
|------|-----------|------|-----|-------------|------|----------|----------|
|      |           |      |     |             |      |          |          |
|      |           |      |     |             |      |          |          |
|      |           |      |     |             |      |          |          |
|      |           |      |     |             |      |          |          |
|      |           |      |     |             |      |          |          |
|      |           |      |     |             |      |          |          |
|      |           |      |     |             |      |          |          |
|      |           |      |     |             |      |          |          |
|      |           |      |     |             |      |          |          |
|      |           |      |     |             |      |          |          |
|      |           |      |     |             |      |          |          |
|      |           |      |     |             |      |          |          |
|      |           |      |     |             |      |          |          |

# Please complete for all use of extra-glottic devices
(Use codes in index where indicated*)

| Date | EGD type* | Case | Age | Indication* | Size | Attempts | Confirm* |
|------|-----------|------|-----|-------------|------|----------|----------|
|      |           |      |     |             |      |          |          |
|      |           |      |     |             |      |          |          |
|      |           |      |     |             |      |          |          |
|      |           |      |     |             |      |          |          |
|      |           |      |     |             |      |          |          |
|      |           |      |     |             |      |          |          |
|      |           |      |     |             |      |          |          |
|      |           |      |     |             |      |          |          |
|      |           |      |     |             |      |          |          |
|      |           |      |     |             |      |          |          |
|      |           |      |     |             |      |          |          |
|      |           |      |     |             |      |          |          |
|      |           |      |     |             |      |          |          |

## Please complete for all use of extra-glottic devices
(Use codes in index where indicated*)

| Date | EGD type* | Case | Age | Indication* | Size | Attempts | Confirm* |
|------|-----------|------|-----|-------------|------|----------|----------|
|      |           |      |     |             |      |          |          |
|      |           |      |     |             |      |          |          |
|      |           |      |     |             |      |          |          |
|      |           |      |     |             |      |          |          |
|      |           |      |     |             |      |          |          |
|      |           |      |     |             |      |          |          |
|      |           |      |     |             |      |          |          |
|      |           |      |     |             |      |          |          |
|      |           |      |     |             |      |          |          |
|      |           |      |     |             |      |          |          |
|      |           |      |     |             |      |          |          |
|      |           |      |     |             |      |          |          |
|      |           |      |     |             |      |          |          |
|      |           |      |     |             |      |          |          |

# Please complete for all ET intubation attempts for which you were the intubator or assistant

(Use codes in index where indicated*)

| Date | INT/ASS | Case | Indication* | DL/VL* | View* | Bougie | Attempts | Confirm* |
|------|---------|------|-------------|--------|-------|--------|----------|----------|
|      |         |      |             |        |       |        |          |          |
|      |         |      |             |        |       |        |          |          |
|      |         |      |             |        |       |        |          |          |
|      |         |      |             |        |       |        |          |          |
|      |         |      |             |        |       |        |          |          |
|      |         |      |             |        |       |        |          |          |
|      |         |      |             |        |       |        |          |          |
|      |         |      |             |        |       |        |          |          |
|      |         |      |             |        |       |        |          |          |
|      |         |      |             |        |       |        |          |          |
|      |         |      |             |        |       |        |          |          |
|      |         |      |             |        |       |        |          |          |

**Please complete for all ET intubation attempts for which you were the intubator or assistant**

(Use codes in index where indicated*)

| Date | INT/ASS | Case | Indication* | DL/VL* | View* | Bougie | Attempts | Confirm* |
|------|---------|------|-------------|--------|-------|--------|----------|----------|
|      |         |      |             |        |       |        |          |          |
|      |         |      |             |        |       |        |          |          |
|      |         |      |             |        |       |        |          |          |
|      |         |      |             |        |       |        |          |          |
|      |         |      |             |        |       |        |          |          |
|      |         |      |             |        |       |        |          |          |
|      |         |      |             |        |       |        |          |          |
|      |         |      |             |        |       |        |          |          |
|      |         |      |             |        |       |        |          |          |
|      |         |      |             |        |       |        |          |          |
|      |         |      |             |        |       |        |          |          |
|      |         |      |             |        |       |        |          |          |

# Please complete for all ET intubation attempts for which you were the intubator or assistant

(Use codes in index where indicated*)

| Date | INT/ASS | Case | Indication* | DL/VL* | View* | Bougie | Attempts | Confirm* |
|------|---------|------|-------------|--------|-------|--------|----------|----------|
|      |         |      |             |        |       |        |          |          |
|      |         |      |             |        |       |        |          |          |
|      |         |      |             |        |       |        |          |          |
|      |         |      |             |        |       |        |          |          |
|      |         |      |             |        |       |        |          |          |
|      |         |      |             |        |       |        |          |          |
|      |         |      |             |        |       |        |          |          |
|      |         |      |             |        |       |        |          |          |
|      |         |      |             |        |       |        |          |          |
|      |         |      |             |        |       |        |          |          |
|      |         |      |             |        |       |        |          |          |
|      |         |      |             |        |       |        |          |          |

**Please complete for all ET intubation attempts for which you were the intubator or assistant**
(Use codes in index where indicated*)

| Date | INT/ASS | Case | Indication* | DL/VL* | View* | Bougie | Attempts | Confirm* |
|------|---------|------|-------------|--------|-------|--------|----------|----------|
|      |         |      |             |        |       |        |          |          |
|      |         |      |             |        |       |        |          |          |
|      |         |      |             |        |       |        |          |          |
|      |         |      |             |        |       |        |          |          |
|      |         |      |             |        |       |        |          |          |
|      |         |      |             |        |       |        |          |          |
|      |         |      |             |        |       |        |          |          |
|      |         |      |             |        |       |        |          |          |
|      |         |      |             |        |       |        |          |          |
|      |         |      |             |        |       |        |          |          |
|      |         |      |             |        |       |        |          |          |
|      |         |      |             |        |       |        |          |          |

## Please complete for all ET intubation attempts for which you were the intubator or assistant

(Use codes in index where indicated*)

| Date | INT/ASS | Case | Indication* | DL/VL* | View* | Bougie | Attempts | Confirm* |
|------|---------|------|-------------|--------|-------|--------|----------|----------|
|      |         |      |             |        |       |        |          |          |
|      |         |      |             |        |       |        |          |          |
|      |         |      |             |        |       |        |          |          |
|      |         |      |             |        |       |        |          |          |
|      |         |      |             |        |       |        |          |          |
|      |         |      |             |        |       |        |          |          |
|      |         |      |             |        |       |        |          |          |
|      |         |      |             |        |       |        |          |          |
|      |         |      |             |        |       |        |          |          |
|      |         |      |             |        |       |        |          |          |
|      |         |      |             |        |       |        |          |          |
|      |         |      |             |        |       |        |          |          |

## Please complete for all use of other clinical skills
(Use codes in index where indicated*)

| Date | Skill | Case | Age | Indication* | Site | Kit used | Confirm* |
|------|-------|------|-----|-------------|------|----------|----------|
|      |       |      |     |             |      |          |          |
|      |       |      |     |             |      |          |          |
|      |       |      |     |             |      |          |          |
|      |       |      |     |             |      |          |          |
|      |       |      |     |             |      |          |          |
|      |       |      |     |             |      |          |          |
|      |       |      |     |             |      |          |          |
|      |       |      |     |             |      |          |          |
|      |       |      |     |             |      |          |          |
|      |       |      |     |             |      |          |          |
|      |       |      |     |             |      |          |          |
|      |       |      |     |             |      |          |          |